This Journal Belongs To:

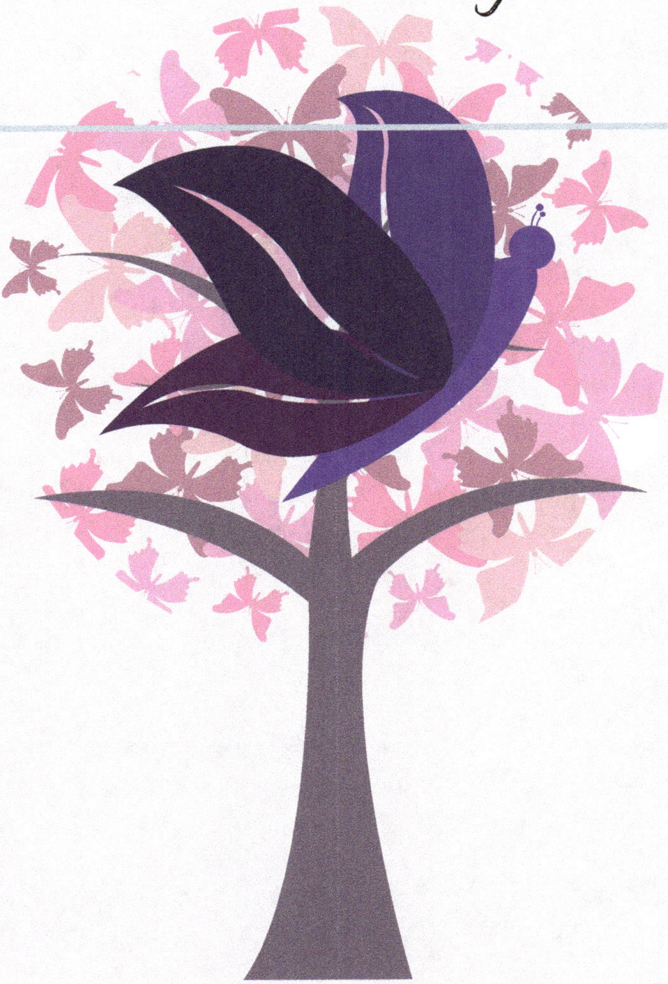

The Need For Change

In a conversation with a mentee, they asked why God has not yet changed them desp[ite] the continued prayers.
A change of heart is their desire
A change of mind or mindset
A change of attitude
Change of habits
The list seems to go on...

Yet, the question I presented was how many opportunities did God place before them [to] begin taking steps to walk into the light of day and make even the slightest change or s[ign] that change was possible, but they decided to stay where they were?
How often or how many times did God present himself as an answer, but they turne[d] away because they wanted or expected things to only go according to their understanding, yet prayed for a change of mind and heart?
How can we expect this great move from God yet be so unwilling to work in tandem w[ith] him?

Perhaps we lack the faith we need to trust and believe that he will answer us in the fir[st] place. Maybe the initial change we must make is our belief. For how can we ask of something yet be so unwilling, uncooperative in the expected outcome?
If change is what you seek, then expect what you desire, then expect it to come in way[s] that differ from what you are used to. Be willing to answer the call and cooperate whe[n] needed.

Be ready to make the change, take part in the change you seek rather than a passive stance that only leads to further diminished faith that, frankly, you cannot blame Go[d] for.

If you seek him for something, at least be willing to say "YES" to what you are seeking h[im] for. Then become the change you want to see, working in unity with the King of kings[.]

CHANGE IS WHAT WE SEEK,
YET WHEN THE OPPORTUNITY
PRESENTS,
DO WE TAKE THE NECESSARY STEPS
TO ACTUALLY BEGIN
MAKE THE CHANGE WE DESIRE?

EVERY GREAT LEADER HAS A VOICE. A MESSAGE THAT NEEDS TO BE HEARD FOR THE TIME THEY ARE IN. THE MESSAGES THEY CARRY CAN IGNITE CHANGE, PEACE, AND MAY EVEN SPARK A FIRE TO IGNITE OTHER LEADERS TO ARISE.

As are the owners of the space in which we live, we can choose to create a space that invites peace & harmony or create a space that continues to promote chaos & dysfunction

Want to make a difference?
Change starts with you!
Change your perspective
Change your attitude
Change how you treat others

CHANGE IS WHAT WE SEEK,
YET WHEN THE OPPORTUNITY
PRESENTS,
WE TAKE THE NECESSARY STEPS
TO ACTUALLY BEGIN
MAKE THE CHANGE WE DESIRE?

EVERY GREAT LEADER HAS A VOICE, A MESSAGE THAT NEEDS TO BE HEARD FOR THE TIME THEY ARE IN. THE MESSAGES THEY CARRY CAN IGNITE CHANGE, PEACE, AND MAY EVEN SPARK A FIRE TO IGNITE OTHER LEADERS TO ARISE.

We are the owners of the space in which we live, we can choose to create a space that invites peace & harmony or create a space that continues to promote chaos & dysfunction

Want to make a difference?
Change starts with you!
Change your perspective
Change your attitude
Change how you treat others

Fresh Manna
Shawanda R. Randolph

CHANGE IS WHAT WE SEEK. YET WHEN THE OPPORTUNITY PRESENTS, WE TAKE THE NECESSARY STEPS TO ACTUALLY BEGIN MAKE THE CHANGE WE DESIRE?

EVERY GREAT LEADER HAS A VOICE, A MESSAGE THAT NEEDS TO BE HEARD FOR THE TIME THEY ARE IN. THE MESSAGES THEY CARRY CAN IGNITE CHANGE, PEACE, AND MAY EVEN SPARK A FIRE TO IGNITE OTHER LEADERS TO ARISE.

we are the owners of the space in which we live. we can choose to create a space that invites peace & harmony or create a space that continues to promote chaos & dysfunction

Want to make a difference?
Change starts with you!
Change your perspective
Change your attitude
Change how you treat others

CHANGE IS WHAT WE SEEK,
YET WHEN THE OPPORTUNITY PRESENTS,
WE TAKE THE NECESSARY STEPS
TO ACTUALLY BEGIN
MAKE THE CHANGE WE DESIRE?

EVERY GREAT LEADER HAS A VOICE, A MESSAGE THAT NEEDS TO BE HEARD FOR THE TIME THEY ARE IN. THE MESSAGES THEY CARRY CAN IGNITE CHANGE, PEACE, AND MAY EVEN SPARK A FIRE TO IGNITE OTHER LEADERS TO ARISE.

As are the owners of the space in which we live, we can choose to [cre]ate a space that invites peace & [h]armony or create a space that continues to promote chaos & dysfunction

Want to make a difference?
Change starts with you!
Change your perspective
Change your attitude
Change how you treat others

Fresh Manna
Shawanda R. Randolph

CHANGE IS WHAT WE SEEK.
YET WHEN THE OPPORTUNITY
PRESENTS,
WE TAKE THE NECESSARY STEPS
TO ACTUALLY BEGIN
MAKE THE CHANGE WE DESIRE?

EVERY GREAT LEADER HAS A VOICE, A MESSAGE THAT NEEDS TO BE HEARD FOR THE TIME THEY ARE IN. THE MESSAGES THEY CARRY CAN IGNITE CHANGE, PEACE, AND MAY EVEN SPARK A FIRE TO IGNITE OTHER LEADERS TO ARISE.

We are the owners of the space in which we live, we can choose to create a space that invites peace & harmony or create a space that continues to promote chaos & dysfunction

Want to make a difference?
Change starts with you!
Change your perspective
Change your attitude
Change how you treat others

Fresh Manna
Shawanda R. Randolph

CHANGE IS WHAT WE SEEK. YET WHEN THE OPPORTUNITY PRESENTS, WE TAKE THE NECESSARY STEPS TO ACTUALLY BEGIN MAKE THE CHANGE WE DESIRE?

EVERY GREAT LEADER HAS A VOICE, A MESSAGE THAT NEEDS TO BE HEARD FOR THE TIME THEY ARE IN. THE MESSAGES THEY CARRY CAN IGNITE CHANGE, PEACE, AND MAY EVEN SPARK A FIRE TO IGNITE OTHER LEADERS TO ARISE.

We are the owners of the space in which we live, we can choose to create a space that invites peace & harmony or create a space that continues to promote chaos & dysfunction

Want to make a difference?
Change starts with you!
Change your perspective
Change your attitude
Change how you treat others

Fresh Manna
Shawanda R. Randolph

CHANGE IS WHAT WE SEEK,
YET WHEN THE OPPORTUNITY PRESENTS,
WE TAKE THE NECESSARY STEPS TO ACTUALLY BEGIN
MAKE THE CHANGE WE DESIRE?

EVERY GREAT LEADER HAS A VOICE, A MESSAGE THAT NEEDS TO BE HEARD FOR THE TIME THEY ARE IN. THE MESSAGES THEY CARRY CAN IGNITE CHANGE, PEACE, AND MAY EVEN SPARK A FIRE TO IGNITE OTHER LEADERS TO ARISE.

[We] are the owners of the space in [w]hich we live, we can choose to [cre]ate a space that invites peace & [h]armony or create a space that continues to promote chaos & dysfunction

Want to make a difference?
Change starts with you!
Change your perspective
Change your attitude
Change how you treat others

Fresh Manna
Shawonda R. Randolph

CHANGE IS WHAT WE SEEK,
YET WHEN THE OPPORTUNITY
PRESENTS,
WE TAKE THE NECESSARY STEPS
TO ACTUALLY BEGIN
MAKE THE CHANGE WE DESIRE?

EVERY GREAT LEADER HAS A VOICE, A MESSAGE THAT NEEDS TO BE HEARD FOR THE TIME THEY ARE IN. THE MESSAGES THEY CARRY CAN IGNITE CHANGE, PEACE, AND MAY EVEN SPARK A FIRE TO IGNITE OTHER LEADERS TO ARISE.

We are the owners of the space in which we live, we can choose to create a space that invites peace & harmony or create a space that continues to promote chaos & dysfunction

Want to make a difference?
Change starts with you!
Change your perspective
Change your attitude
Change how you treat others

Fresh Manna
Shawanda R. Randolph

CHANGE IS WHAT WE SEEK, YET WHEN THE OPPORTUNITY PRESENTS, WE TAKE THE NECESSARY STEPS TO ACTUALLY BEGIN MAKE THE CHANGE WE DESIRE?

_____
_____
_____
_____
_____
_____
_____
_____
_____
_____
_____
_____
_____
_____
_____
_____
_____
_____
_____
_____
_____
_____
_____
_____
_____
_____
_____
_____
_____
_____
_____
_____

EVERY GREAT LEADER HAS A VOICE, A MESSAGE THAT NEEDS TO BE HEARD FOR THE TIME THEY ARE IN. THE MESSAGES THEY CARRY CAN IGNITE CHANGE, PEACE, AND MAY EVEN SPARK A FIRE TO IGNITE OTHER LEADERS TO ARISE.

We are the owners of the space in which we live. we can choose to create a space that invites peace & harmony or create a space that continues to promote chaos & dysfunction

Want to make a difference?
Change starts with you!
Change your perspective
Change your attitude
Change how you treat others

**CHANGE IS WHAT WE SEEK,
YET WHEN THE OPPORTUNITY
PRESENTS,
WE TAKE THE NECESSARY STEPS
TO ACTUALLY BEGIN
MAKE THE CHANGE WE DESIRE?**

EVERY GREAT LEADER HAS A VOICE, A MESSAGE THAT NEEDS TO BE HEARD FOR THE TIME THEY ARE IN. THE MESSAGES THEY CARRY CAN IGNITE CHANGE, PEACE, AND MAY EVEN SPARK A FIRE TO IGNITE OTHER LEADERS TO ARISE.

> We are the owners of the space in which we live, we can choose to create a space that invites peace & harmony or create a space that continues to promote chaos & dysfunction

Want to make a difference?
Change starts with you!
Change your perspective
Change your attitude
Change how you treat others

Fresh Manna
Shawonda R. Randolph

CHANGE IS WHAT WE SEEK,
YET WHEN THE OPPORTUNITY
PRESENTS,
WE TAKE THE NECESSARY STEPS
TO ACTUALLY BEGIN
MAKE THE CHANGE WE DESIRE?

EVERY GREAT LEADER HAS A VOICE, A MESSAGE THAT NEEDS TO BE HEARD FOR THE TIME THEY ARE IN. THE MESSAGES THEY CARRY CAN IGNITE CHANGE, PEACE, AND MAY EVEN SPARK A FIRE TO IGNITE OTHER LEADERS TO ARISE.

We are the owners of the space in which we live, we can choose to create a space that invites peace & harmony or create a space that continues to promote chaos & dysfunction

Want to make a difference?
Change starts with you!
Change your perspective
Change your attitude
Change how you treat others

Fresh Manna
Shawanda R. Randolph

CHANGE IS WHAT WE SEEK, YET WHEN THE OPPORTUNITY PRESENTS, WE TAKE THE NECESSARY STEPS TO ACTUALLY BEGIN MAKE THE CHANGE WE DESIRE?

> EVERY GREAT LEADER HAS A VOICE, A MESSAGE THAT NEEDS TO BE HEARD FOR THE TIME THEY ARE IN. THE MESSAGES THEY CARRY CAN IGNITE CHANGE, PEACE, AND MAY EVEN SPARK A FIRE TO IGNITE OTHER LEADERS TO ARISE.

We are the owners of the space in which we live, we can choose to create a space that invites peace & harmony or create a space that continues to promote chaos & dysfunction

Want to make a difference?
Change starts with you!
Change your perspective
Change your attitude
Change how you treat others

Fresh Manna
Shawanda R. Randolph

CHANGE IS WHAT WE SEEK,
YET WHEN THE OPPORTUNITY
PRESENTS,
WE TAKE THE NECESSARY STEPS
TO ACTUALLY BEGIN
MAKE THE CHANGE WE DESIRE?

EVERY GREAT LEADER HAS A VOICE, A MESSAGE THAT NEEDS TO BE HEARD FOR THE TIME THEY ARE IN. THE MESSAGES THEY CARRY CAN IGNITE CHANGE, PEACE, AND MAY EVEN SPARK A FIRE TO IGNITE OTHER LEADERS TO ARISE.

> As are the owners of the space in which we live, we can choose to create a space that invites peace & harmony or create a space that continues to promote chaos & dysfunction

Want to make a difference?
Change starts with you!
Change your perspective
Change your attitude
Change how you treat others

Fresh Manna
Shawonda R. Randolph

CHANGE IS WHAT WE SEEK,
YET WHEN THE OPPORTUNITY
PRESENTS,
WE TAKE THE NECESSARY STEPS
TO ACTUALLY BEGIN
MAKE THE CHANGE WE DESIRE?

EVERY GREAT LEADER HAS A VOICE, A MESSAGE THAT NEEDS TO BE HEARD FOR THE TIME THEY ARE IN. THE MESSAGES THEY CARRY CAN IGNITE CHANGE, PEACE, AND MAY EVEN SPARK A FIRE TO IGNITE OTHER LEADERS TO ARISE.

[We] are the owners of the space in which we live, we can choose to [cre]ate a space that invites peace & [h]armony or create a space that continues to promote chaos & dysfunction

Want to make a difference?
Change starts with you!
Change your perspective
Change your attitude
Change how you treat others

CHANGE IS WHAT WE SEEK. YET WHEN THE OPPORTUNITY PRESENTS, WE TAKE THE NECESSARY STEPS TO ACTUALLY BEGIN MAKE THE CHANGE WE DESIRE?

EVERY GREAT LEADER HAS A VOICE, A MESSAGE THAT NEEDS TO BE HEARD FOR THE TIME THEY ARE IN. THE MESSAGES THEY CARRY CAN IGNITE CHANGE, PEACE, AND MAY EVEN SPARK A FIRE TO IGNITE OTHER LEADERS TO ARISE.

We are the owners of the space in which we live, we can choose to create a space that invites peace & harmony or create a space that continues to promote chaos & dysfunction

Want to make a difference?
Change starts with you!
Change your perspective
Change your attitude
Change how you treat others

Fresh Manna
Shawanda R. Randolph

CHANGE IS WHAT WE SEEK,
YET WHEN THE OPPORTUNITY
PRESENTS,
WE TAKE THE NECESSARY STEPS
TO ACTUALLY BEGIN
MAKE THE CHANGE WE DESIRE?

EVERY GREAT LEADER HAS A VOICE, A MESSAGE THAT NEEDS TO BE HEARD FOR THE TIME THEY ARE IN. THE MESSAGES THEY CARRY CAN IGNITE CHANGE, PEACE, AND MAY EVEN SPARK A FIRE TO IGNITE OTHER LEADERS TO ARISE.

...e are the owners of the space in which we live, we can choose to ...ate a space that invites peace & ...armony or create a space that continues to promote chaos & dysfunction

Want to make a difference?
Change starts with you!
Change your perspective
Change your attitude
Change how you treat others

Fresh Manna
Shawanda R. Randolph

CHANGE IS WHAT WE SEEK, YET WHEN THE OPPORTUNITY PRESENTS, WE TAKE THE NECESSARY STEPS TO ACTUALLY BEGIN MAKE THE CHANGE WE DESIRE?

EVERY GREAT LEADER HAS A VOICE, A MESSAGE THAT NEEDS TO BE HEARD FOR THE TIME THEY ARE IN. THE MESSAGES THEY CARRY CAN IGNITE CHANGE, PEACE, AND MAY EVEN SPARK A FIRE TO IGNITE OTHER LEADERS TO ARISE.

We are the owners of the space in which we live, we can choose to create a space that invites peace & harmony or create a space that continues to promote chaos & dysfunction

Want to make a difference?
Change starts with you!
Change your perspective
Change your attitude
Change how you treat others

Fresh Manna
Shawanda R. Randolph

CHANGE IS WHAT WE SEEK,
YET WHEN THE OPPORTUNITY PRESENTS,
WE TAKE THE NECESSARY STEPS TO ACTUALLY BEGIN
MAKE THE CHANGE WE DESIRE?

EVERY GREAT LEADER HAS A VOICE, A MESSAGE THAT NEEDS TO BE HEARD FOR THE TIME THEY ARE IN. THE MESSAGES THEY CARRY CAN IGNITE CHANGE, PEACE, AND MAY EVEN SPARK A FIRE TO IGNITE OTHER LEADERS TO ARISE.

> We are the owners of the space in which we live, we can choose to create a space that invites peace & harmony or create a space that continues to promote chaos & dysfunction

Want to make a difference?
Change starts with you!
Change your perspective
Change your attitude
Change how you treat others

Fresh Manna
Shawanda R. Randolph

CHANGE IS WHAT WE SEEK, YET WHEN THE OPPORTUNITY PRESENTS, WE TAKE THE NECESSARY STEPS TO ACTUALLY BEGIN MAKE THE CHANGE WE DESIRE?

EVERY GREAT LEADER HAS A VOICE, A MESSAGE THAT NEEDS TO BE HEARD FOR THE TIME THEY ARE IN. THE MESSAGES THEY CARRY CAN IGNITE CHANGE, PEACE, AND MAY EVEN SPARK A FIRE TO IGNITE OTHER LEADERS TO ARISE.

As are the owners of the space in which we live, we can choose to create a space that invites peace & harmony or create a space that continues to promote chaos & dysfunction

Want to make a difference?
Change starts with you!
Change your perspective
Change your attitude
Change how you treat others

CHANGE IS WHAT WE SEEK, YET WHEN THE OPPORTUNITY PRESENTS, WE TAKE THE NECESSARY STEPS TO ACTUALLY BEGIN MAKE THE CHANGE WE DESIRE?

EVERY GREAT LEADER HAS A VOICE, A MESSAGE THAT NEEDS TO BE HEARD FOR THE TIME THEY ARE IN. THE MESSAGES THEY CARRY CAN IGNITE CHANGE, PEACE, AND MAY EVEN SPARK A FIRE TO IGNITE OTHER LEADERS TO ARISE.

e are the owners of the space in which we live, we can choose to create a space that invites peace & harmony or create a space that continues to promote chaos & dysfunction

Want to make a difference?
Change starts with you!
Change your perspective
Change your attitude
Change how you treat others

Fresh Manna
Shawanda R. Randolph

CHANGE IS WHAT WE SEEK,
YET WHEN THE OPPORTUNITY
PRESENTS,
WE TAKE THE NECESSARY STEPS
TO ACTUALLY BEGIN
MAKE THE CHANGE WE DESIRE?

EVERY GREAT LEADER HAS A VOICE, A MESSAGE THAT NEEDS TO BE HEARD FOR THE TIME THEY ARE IN. THE MESSAGES THEY CARRY CAN IGNITE CHANGE, PEACE, AND MAY EVEN SPARK A FIRE TO IGNITE OTHER LEADERS TO ARISE.

We are the owners of the space in which we live, we can choose to create a space that invites peace & harmony or create a space that continues to promote chaos & dysfunction

Want to make a difference?
Change starts with you!
Change your perspective
Change your attitude
Change how you treat others

Fresh Manna
Shawonda R. Randolph

**CHANGE IS WHAT WE SEEK,
YET WHEN THE OPPORTUNITY
PRESENTS,
WE TAKE THE NECESSARY STEPS
TO ACTUALLY BEGIN
MAKE THE CHANGE WE DESIRE?**

EVERY GREAT LEADER HAS A VOICE, A MESSAGE THAT NEEDS TO BE HEARD FOR THE TIME THEY ARE IN. THE MESSAGES THEY CARRY CAN IGNITE CHANGE, PEACE, AND MAY EVEN SPARK A FIRE TO IGNITE OTHER LEADERS TO ARISE.

[We] are the owners of the space in which we live, we can choose to [cre]ate a space that invites peace & [h]armony or create a space that continues to promote chaos & dysfunction

Want to make a difference?
Change starts with you!
Change your perspective
Change your attitude
Change how you treat others

Fresh Manna
Shawanda R. Randolph

CHANGE IS WHAT WE SEEK,
YET WHEN THE OPPORTUNITY
PRESENTS,
WE TAKE THE NECESSARY STEPS
TO ACTUALLY BEGIN
MAKE THE CHANGE WE DESIRE?

EVERY GREAT LEADER HAS A VOICE, A MESSAGE THAT NEEDS TO BE HEARD FOR THE TIME THEY ARE IN. THE MESSAGES THEY CARRY CAN IGNITE CHANGE, PEACE, AND MAY EVEN SPARK A FIRE TO IGNITE OTHER LEADERS TO ARISE.

We are the owners of the space in which we live, we can choose to create a space that invites peace & harmony or create a space that continues to promote chaos & dysfunction

Want to make a difference?
Change starts with you!
Change your perspective
Change your attitude
Change how you treat others

FreshManna
Shawanda R. Randolph

CHANGE IS WHAT WE SEEK, YET WHEN THE OPPORTUNITY PRESENTS, WE TAKE THE NECESSARY STEPS TO ACTUALLY BEGIN MAKE THE CHANGE WE DESIRE?

EVERY GREAT LEADER HAS A VOICE, A MESSAGE THAT NEEDS TO BE HEARD FOR THE TIME THEY ARE IN. THE MESSAGES THEY CARRY CAN IGNITE CHANGE, PEACE, AND MAY EVEN SPARK A FIRE TO IGNITE OTHER LEADERS TO ARISE.

We are the owners of the space in which we live, we can choose to create a space that invites peace & harmony or create a space that continues to promote chaos & dysfunction

Want to make a difference?
Change starts with you!
Change your perspective
Change your attitude
Change how you treat others

Fresh Manna
Shawanda R. Randolph

CHANGE IS WHAT WE SEEK, YET WHEN THE OPPORTUNITY PRESENTS, WE TAKE THE NECESSARY STEPS TO ACTUALLY BEGIN MAKE THE CHANGE WE DESIRE?

EVERY GREAT LEADER HAS A VOICE, A MESSAGE THAT NEEDS TO BE HEARD FOR THE TIME THEY ARE IN. THE MESSAGES THEY CARRY CAN IGNITE CHANGE, PEACE, AND MAY EVEN SPARK A FIRE TO IGNITE OTHER LEADERS TO ARISE.

www.ingramcontent.com/pod-product-compliance
Lightning Source LLC
Chambersburg PA
CBHW071251070526
44583CB00017B/2426